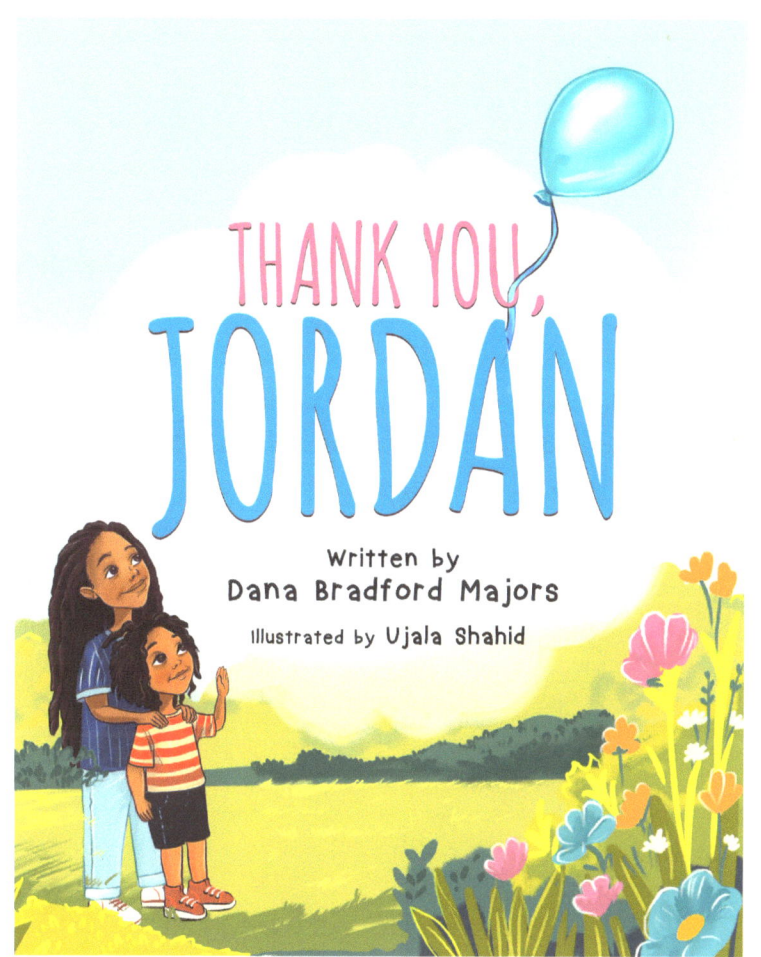

B. MAJORS PUBLISHING

Copyright © 2024 by Dana Bradford-Majors

All rights reserved. This book, or any portion thereof, may not be reproduced or used in any manner whatsoever without the expressed, written permission of the publisher, except for the use of brief quotations in a book review or scholarly journal.

First Edition

ISBN: 979-8-9905207-3-8

United States of America

Illustrated by Ujala Shahid

Layout, Design & Editing by Dana Bradford-Majors

To PJ:
I thank you for the support and memories. Thank you for being there as we navigated this loss.

To Jailyn, Jaleon, and Ayannah:
I'm so proud of you. Losing your brother was not easy, but you all persevered and stepped up to help Mommy through it all! I love you so very much.

To P3; my Rainbow Baby:
I'm so thankful for you! You have made me so proud! I love you so very much!

To my "New Kid", my Surprise Baby, Atreyu:
You never cease to amaze me. I love you so much, New Kid. I'm so happy you are in my life.

To my Baby Boy Jordan:
Not a day goes by that I don't think of you. What you would've looked like, your smile, your personality. I love you so very much. Continue to rest peacefully, Mama's Baby.

Even though I've never met you, I've heard so much.

You would have been only a few months older than me, but you couldn't stay in touch.

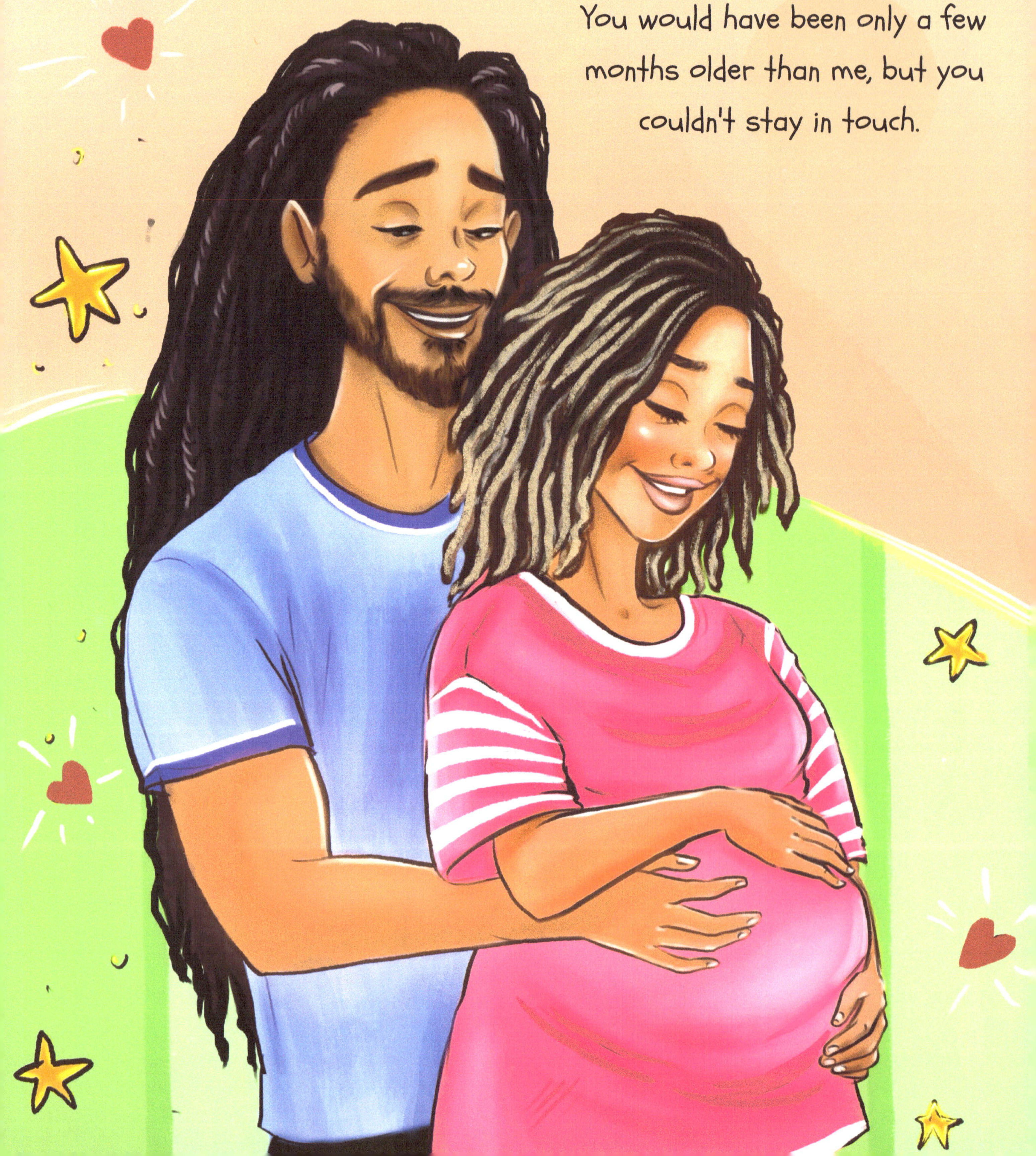

Mom and Dad were just married,
and very happy so it seemed.

Then Mommy found out that she was pregnant with you!
Mommy and Daddy could have screamed!

They beamed with joy! Another child?
They didn't dream it would be so soon.

As Mommy's stomach grew
with you, Daddy swooned!

Weeks would soon pass,
a few months went by, too.

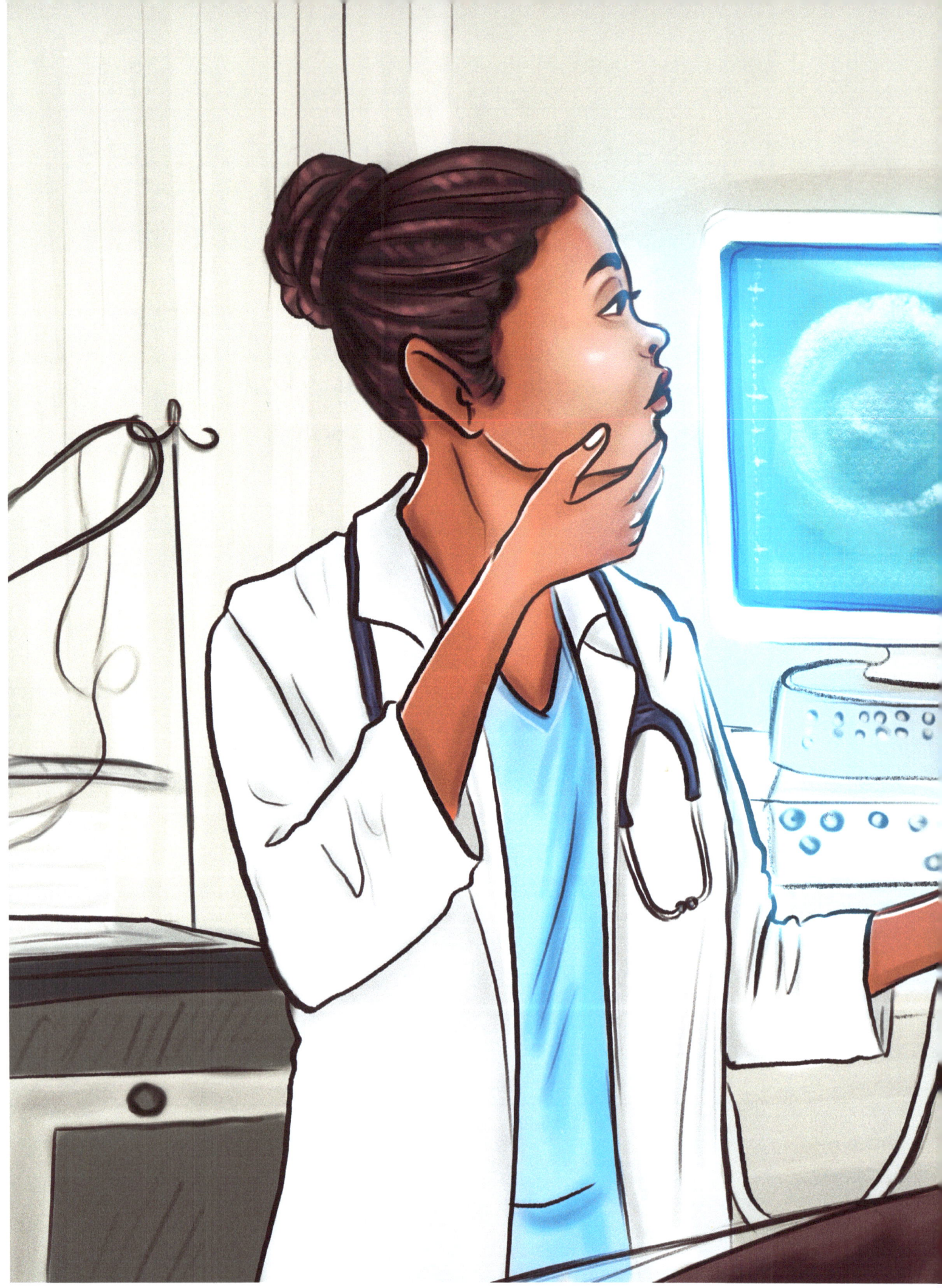

Then, Mommy went to see the doctor to see how big you grew! The doctor's face kind of grimaced; Mommy asked, "Uh oh, what's wrong?"

The doctor told Mommy, "something's not quite right. There's something going on."

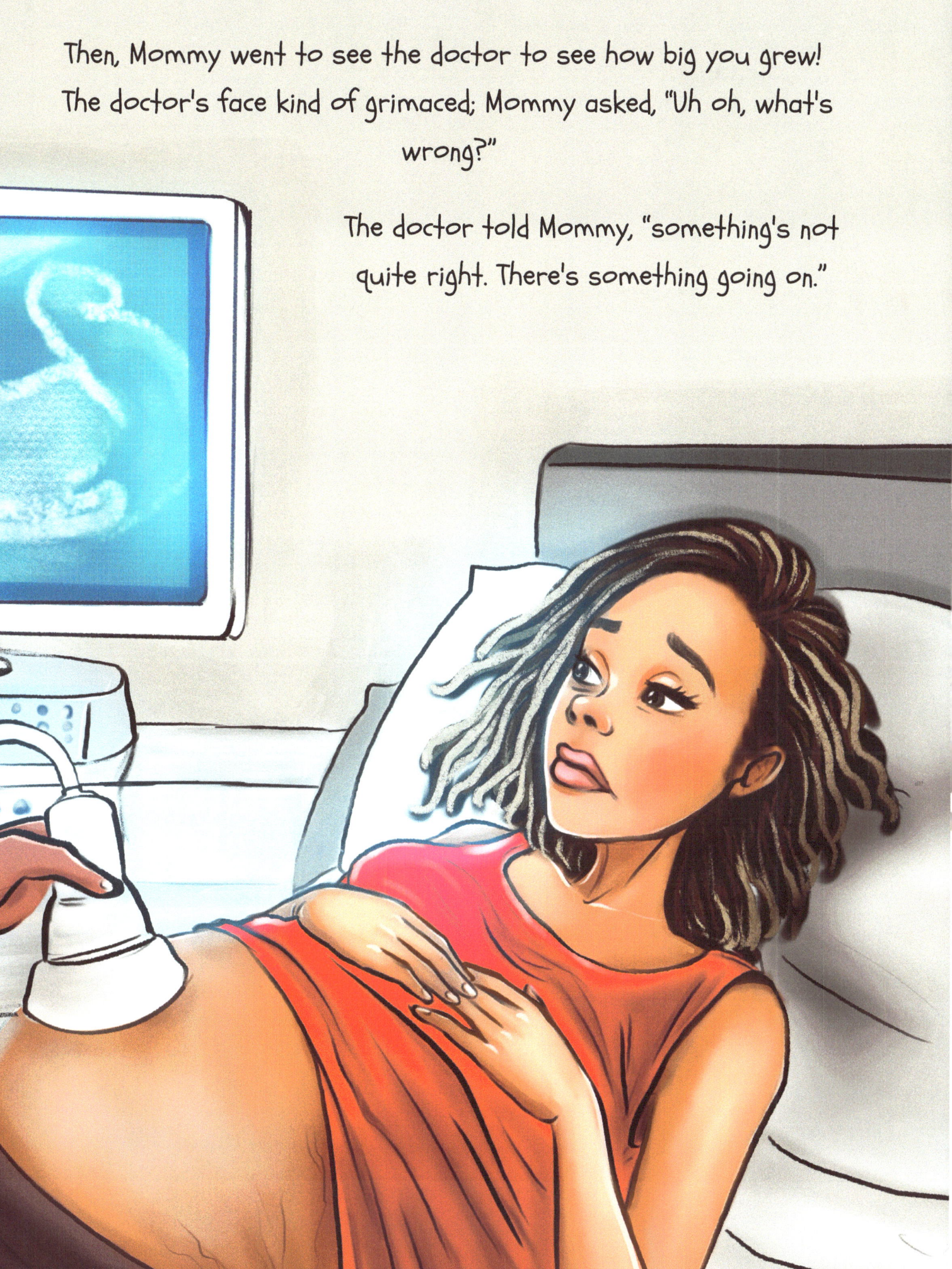

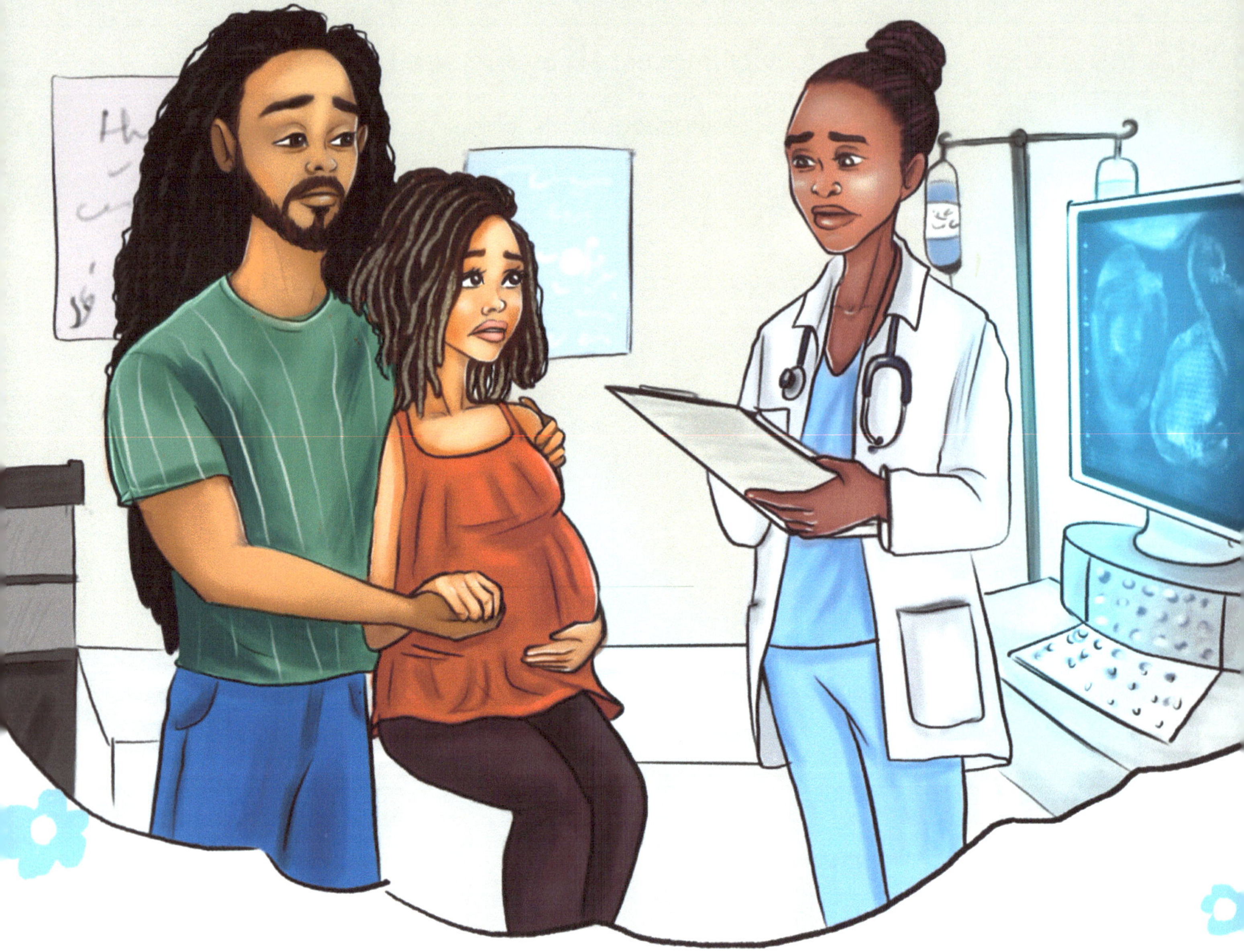

Then, the doctor told Mommy to see a special doctor; the doctor that helps when babies who aren't born yet are sick.

"Maybe this doctor can make you feel better baby," Mommy said, rubbing her tummy. "Maybe something will change, and quick!"

Mommy and Daddy went to the doctor every week, to watch you stretch and grow.

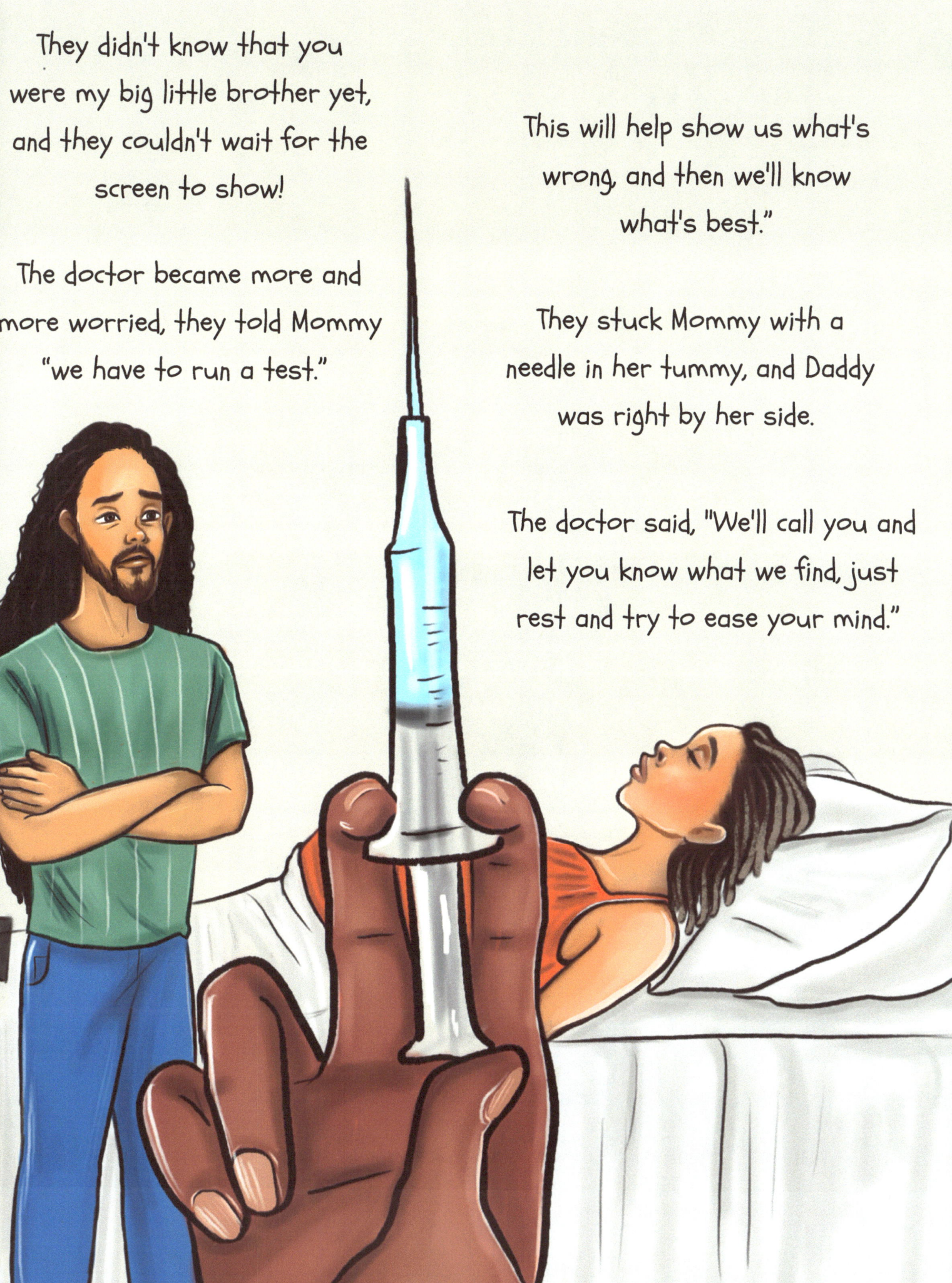

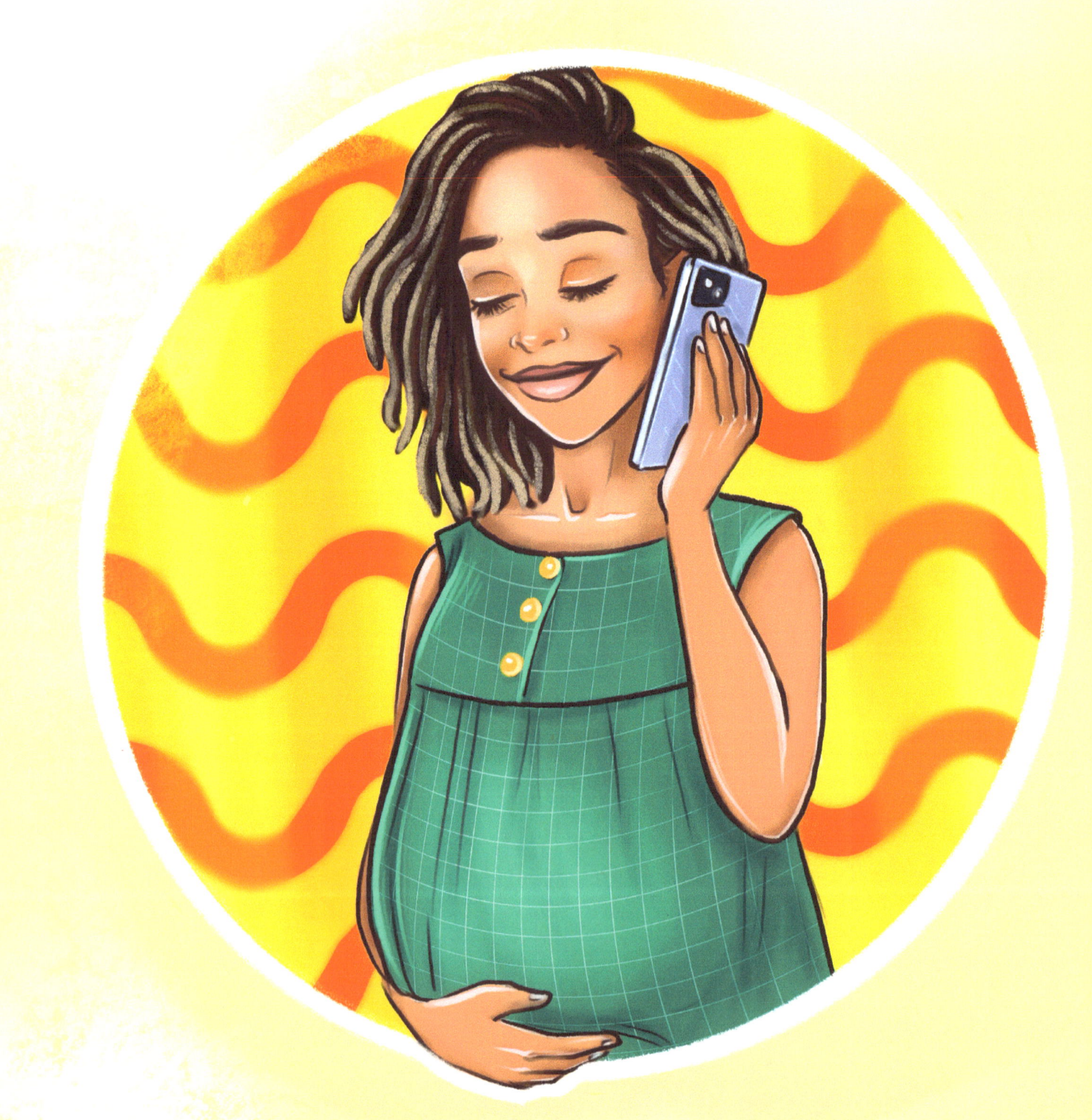

Then, Mommy got a call one day,
and the doctor said "Almost everything is fine!"

"You're having a little boy,
and you'll see him in no time!"

Right there on the spot, Mommy named you Jordan,
and that's now my name, too!

Even though you were sick,
Mommy and Daddy had big plans for you!

The day finally came where Mommy and Daddy would see your face on the screen.

Mommy was lifted on the table, and then hooked up to the machine.

The room was dark and quiet, too quiet so it seemed.

The nurse looked at Mommy and Daddy, very sadly, one tear on her cheek streamed.

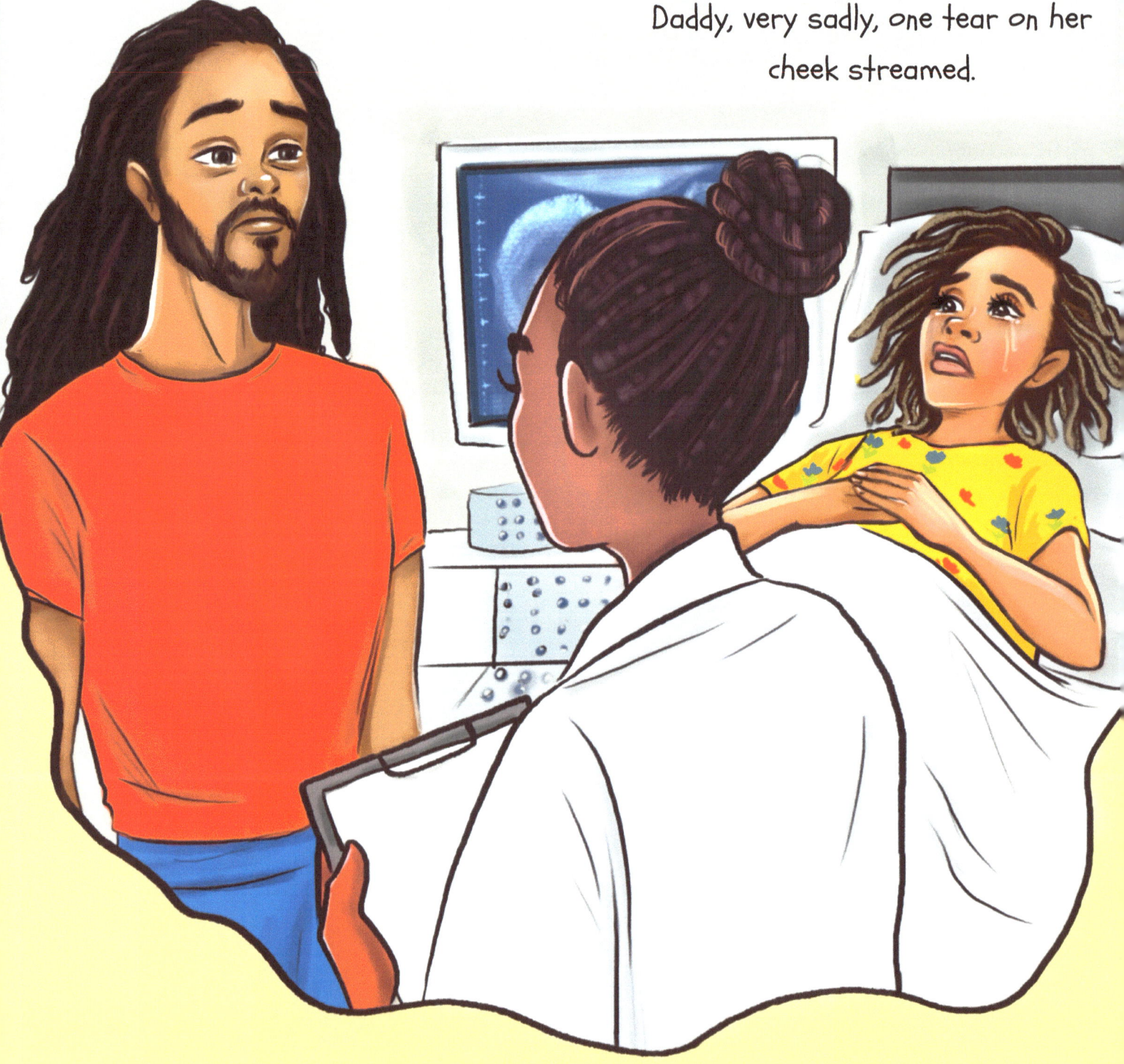

"I'll be right back", said the nurse,
and both Mommy and Daddy were afraid.

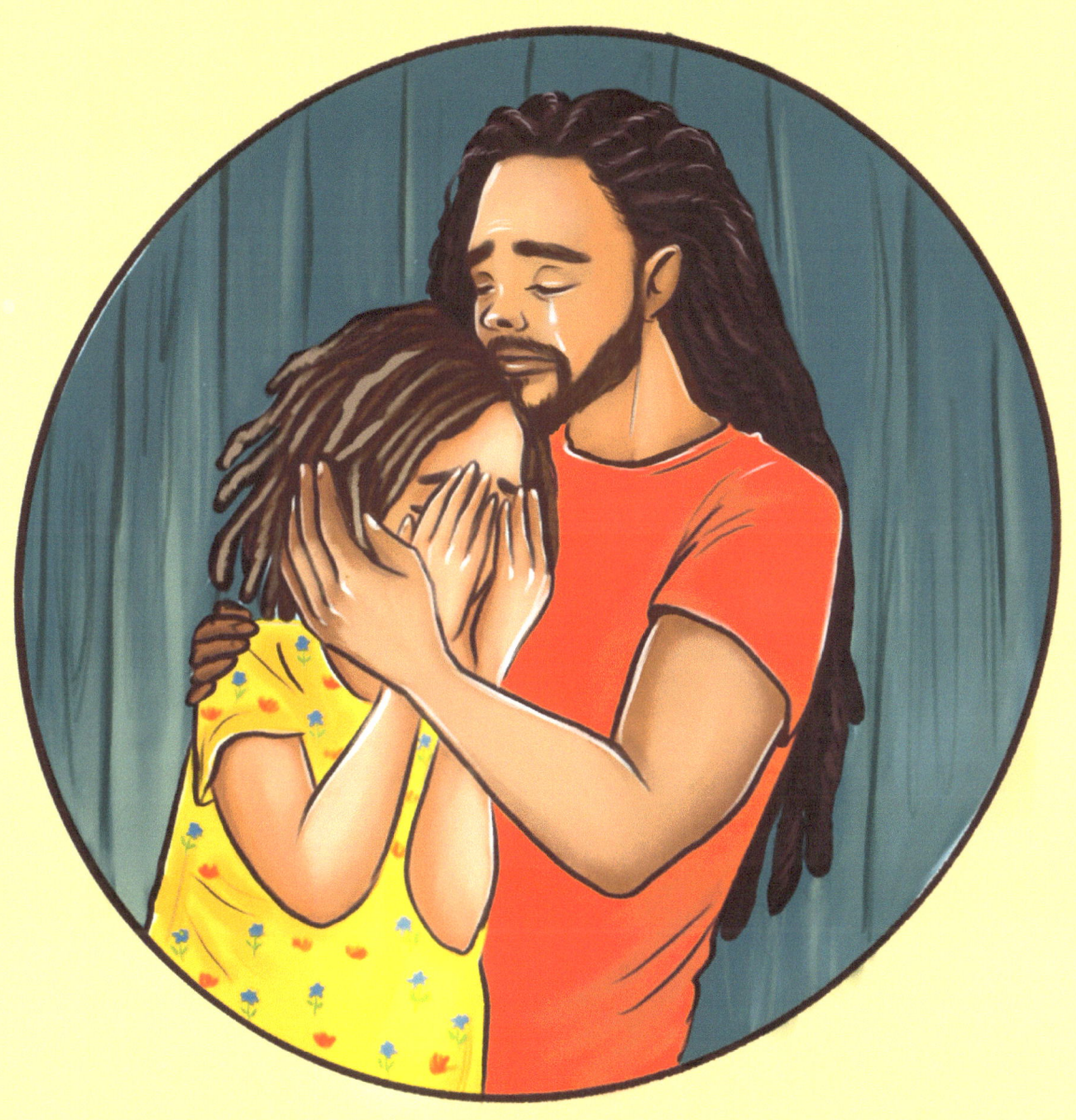

The Doctor came in, looked down and said,
"Jordan's gone." No heartbeat ever played.

Mommy and Daddy cried and were really sad.
They now had an Angel baby; their heartache was really bad.

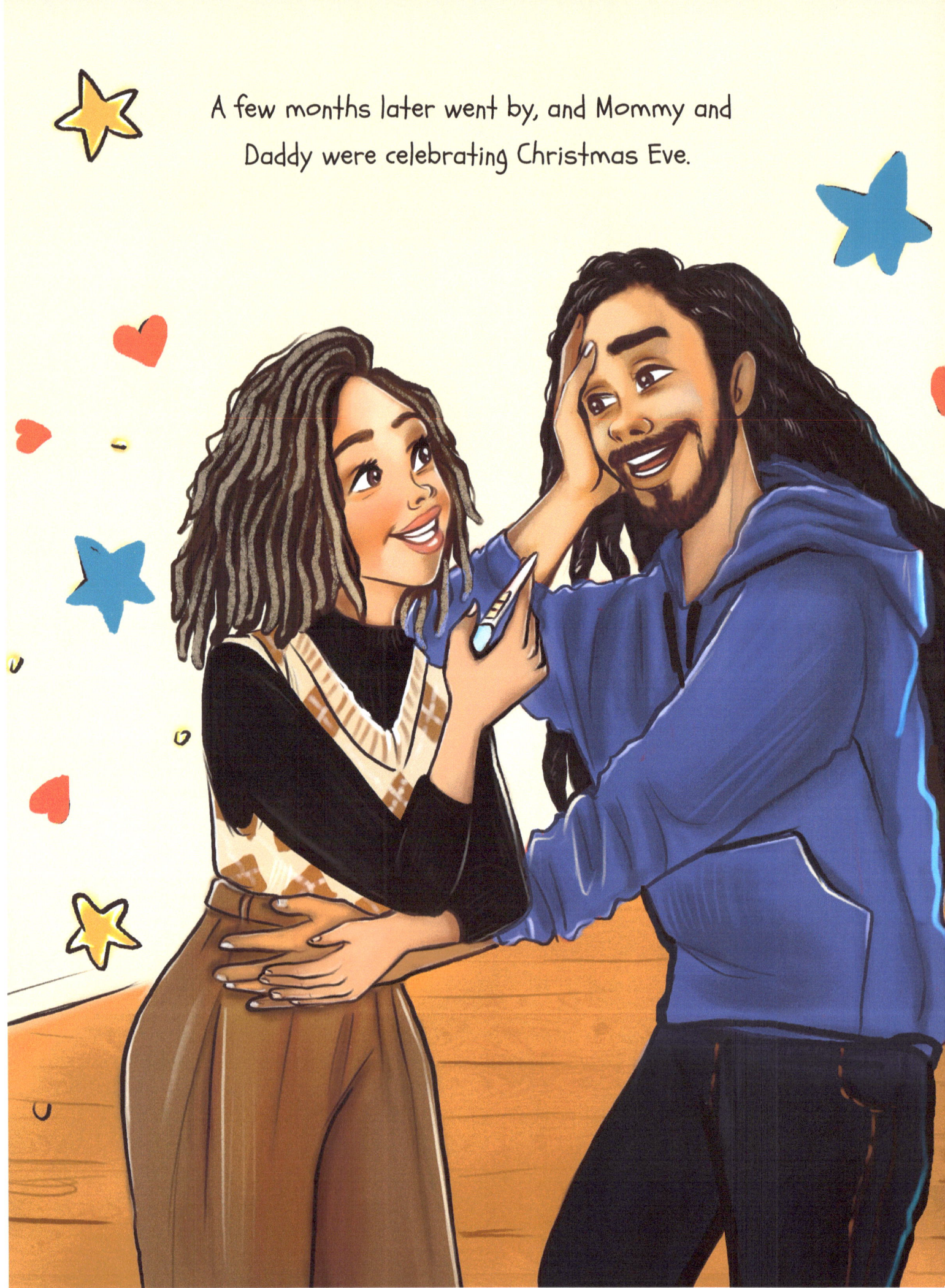
A few months later went by, and Mommy and Daddy were celebrating Christmas Eve.

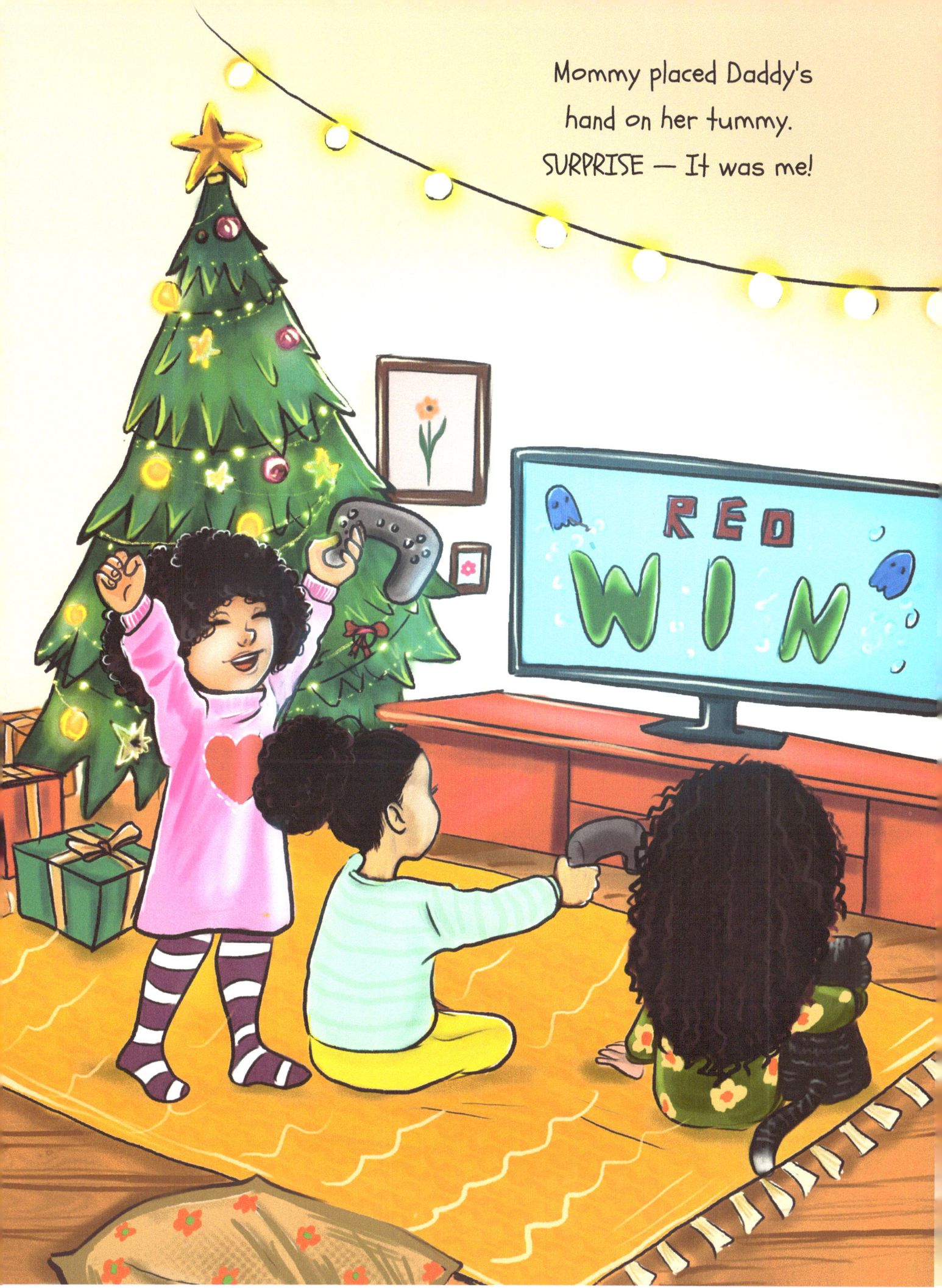

Mommy placed Daddy's hand on her tummy. SURPRISE — It was me!

I came a few months after that,
and then one day I turned three.

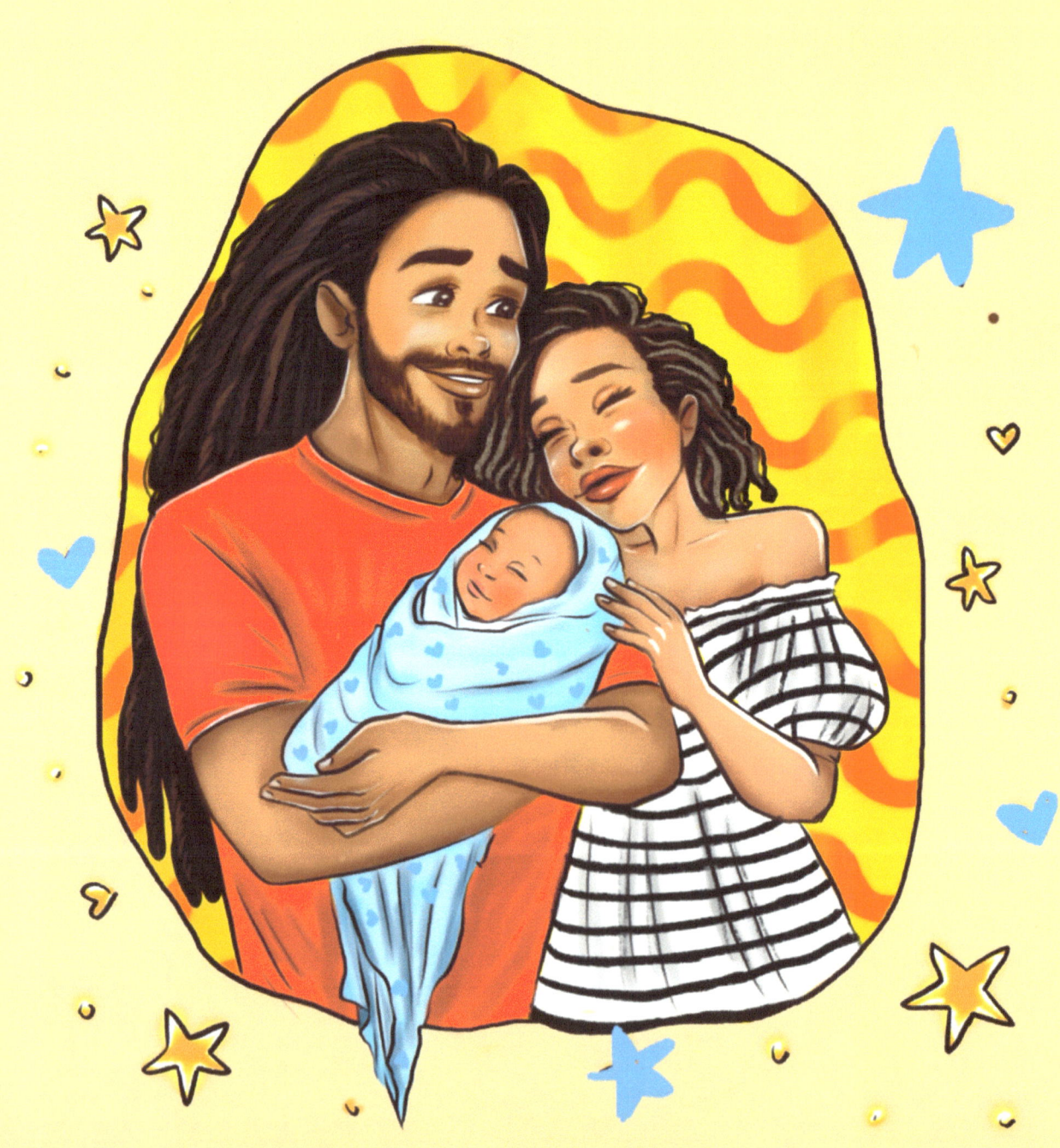

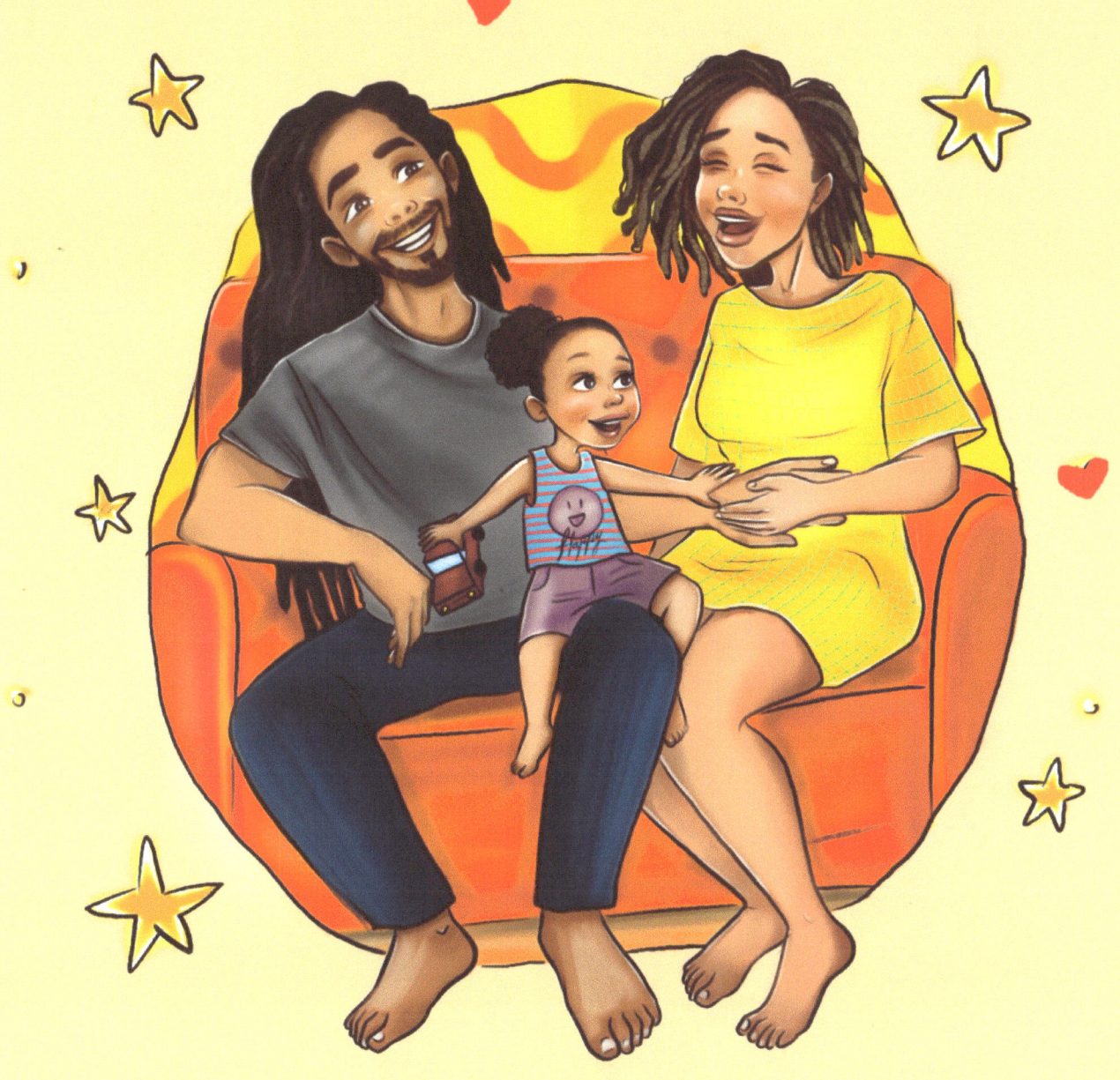

Mommy placed Daddy's hand on her tummy—AGAIN—and New Kid came to be!

Thank you, Jordan, for being my big little brother.
You will always have a place in my heart.

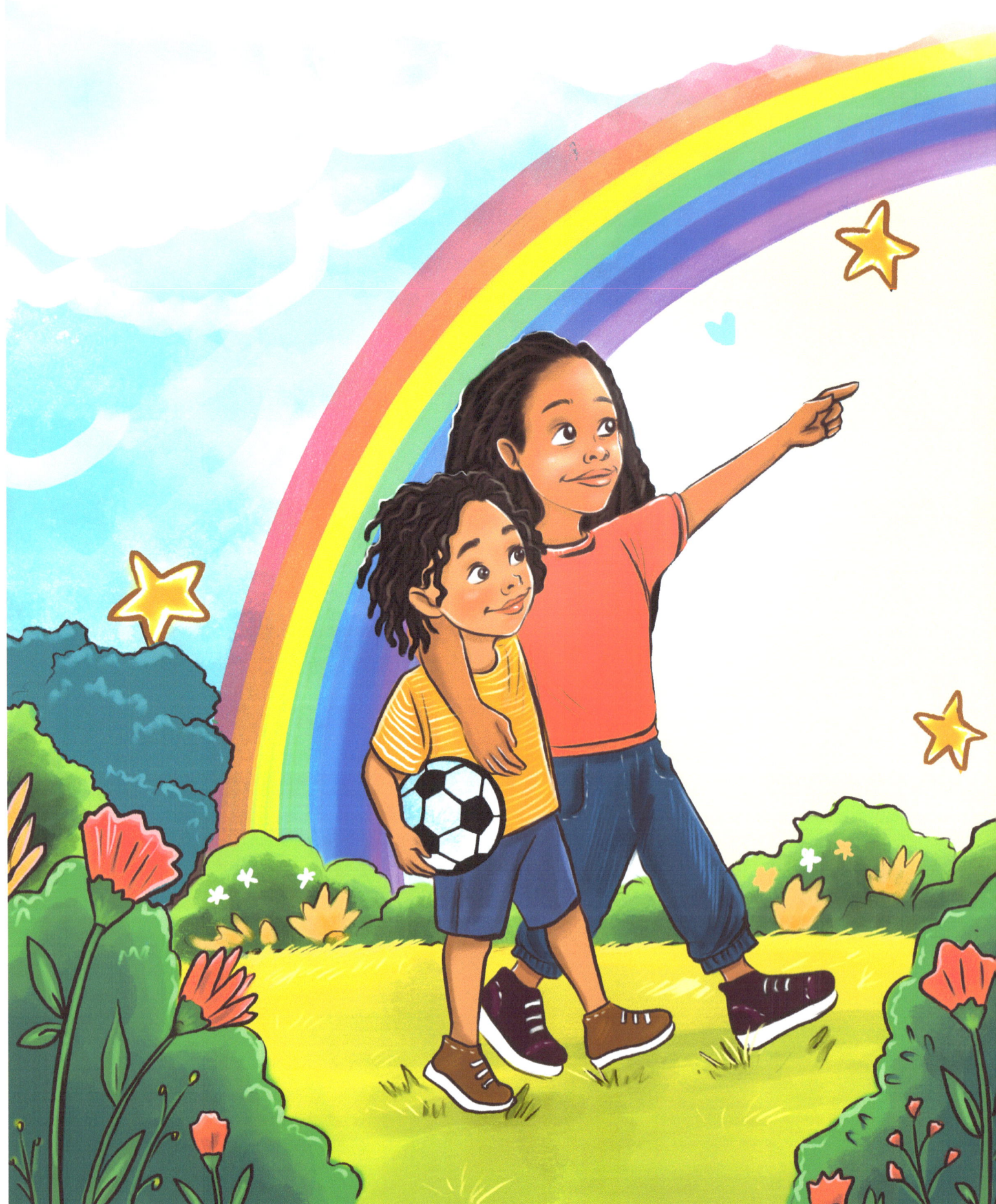

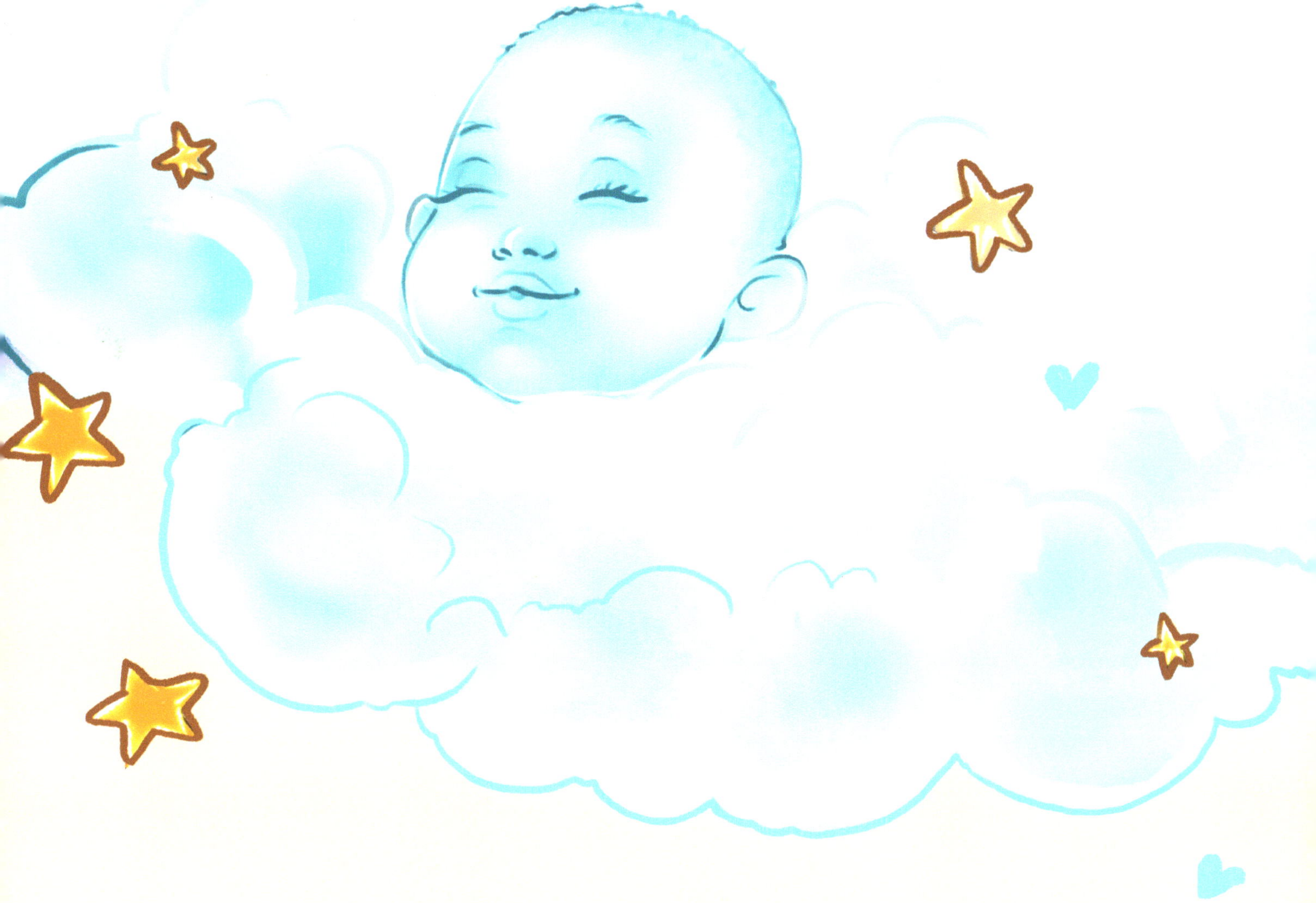

You are Mommy and Daddy's Angel baby,
and you were loved right from the start!

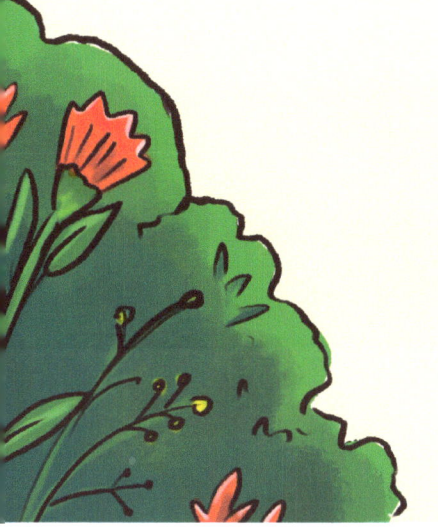

ABOUT THE AUTHOR

Dana Bradford-Majors is the co-author of *Humans Can't Fly*, *...Because Big Boys Aren't Afraid of Outer Space*, *Hey New Kid!* and *A Very Different Butterfly*, in which three of the works are published in the Black Boy Joy series with her sons and co-authors, Pheldon J. Majors, III and Atreyu Majors.

Dana was born and raised in Mississippi and traveled often to New Orleans, Louisiana to visit family and embrace her culture. Dana received a B.A. in English Language Arts from the University of Southern Mississippi, with a minor in Business Technology Education, and a dual M.A. in Workforce Educational Leadership with Advanced Technologies from the prestigious Alcorn State University. Although she has recently shifted her focus to children's book publishing under her own company, B. Majors Publishing, she is currently teaching high school students IT Support . She lives in Indianapolis, Indiana, with her five children of varying personalities, and her dog, Titan.

OTHER TITLES FROM THE "BLACK BOY JOY" SERIES

Humans Can't Fly

¡Los Humanos No Pueden Volar!

...Because Big Boys Aren't Afraid of Outer Space!

Hey New Kid!

¡Hola, Peque!

New Kid and the Day Before Christmas

PREVIOUS WORKS

A Very Different Butterfly

Mrs. Majors is Missing!

FORTHCOMING TITLES FROM B. MAJORS PUBLISHING

Big Boys Have Bad Days, Too!

Finding Mrs. Majors: A Companion Guide to Mrs. Majors is Missing for Social Emotional Learning

www.ingramcontent.com/pod-product-compliance
Lightning Source LLC
Chambersburg PA
CBHW061158030426
42337CB00002B/42